18 Ways to Break into
Medical Coding

Shonda Miles,
CCS, CPC, MBA, CCS-P

www.remote-medical-coding-jobs.com

info@remote-medical-coding-jobs.com

Other books by Author

10 Ways to Write an Ebook every 10 days

101 Success Questions

What I wish I knew before starting an Online Business

Remote Medical Coding Jobs

Tips for Staring an Online Business

How to Love Your Spouse again

How to Double Your Income in 12 Months or less

50 Tips to Jumpstart Your Success

50 Streams of Income

18 Ways to Break into Coding

How to Get the Job You want

21 Ways to Start a Marriage off Right

21 Ways to Make a Blended Family Work

I am for Teens

I am for boys

I am for Girls

Girl Power

Contents

Introduction

"Allow yourself to dream and fantasize about your ideal life; what it would look like, and what it would feel like. Then do something every day to make it a reality!" Brian Tracy

What would it feel like to become a Medical Coder? What does your ideal life look like? Do you want to work from home?

If you really want to be a Medical Coder, then do something every day to become one.

Medical Coding and Billing are both rewarding careers but they do require work. If you got into Medical Coding because you were looking for something easy you are in the wrong field. Medical Coding is work. You have to be detail oriented. You have to love to research. Most importantly you have to be detail oriented.

"Healthcare organizations across the country continue to face severe shortages of qualified coders. The U.S. Department of Labor projects a 22 percent increase – 41,100 openings – in the number of health information technology/management jobs to be filled in the next seven years, with ICD-10 as a major driver for that growth. And, the median annual income of medical coding specialists is more than $50,000."

My name is Shonda Miles. I have a Master's Degree in Business. I have a CPC (Certified Professional Coder) through the American Academy of

Professional Coders, or the AAPC. I have a CCS-P (Certified Coding Specialist-Physician Based) through AHIMA (American Health Information Management Association). I have CCS (Certified Coding Specialist) through AHIMA. This certification is for Inpatient Coders.

I got into coding through a non-traditional route. It's been 15 years. I don't have any formal education in Coding.

I'm going to start off with my story. I was looking for a job that I can do at home. I was having health issues. I was having trouble with my heart, and I needed to find a job that I could do at home. This was around 1999 or 2000. I started a program for medical transcriptionist at a local school here in Shreveport, and I thought, "Okay. This would be great."

I went to school to become a Medical Transcriptionist. I worked for an American Doctor. I thought it was going to be easy to transcribe for him. I knew I didn't want to transcribe for foreign doctors. I knew it was going to be hard to understand them because they talk fast. I thought an American doctor would be perfect. This is exactly what I wanted to do.

It turns out that American doctor's talk just like foreign doctors. They talk fast. They mumble their words. I couldn't understand anything that they were saying. I hated it. What I do remember is that there was one class that I absolutely loved. I wanted to find out more information about it. That class was medical coding. That's how I got started.

I learned enough in that class to get a job in medical coding. I'm going to tell you a real funny story, really quick. The first interview I went on, the first job I tried to get, I went to take the test and I was too ashamed to ask the lady. She gave me the test and said, I don't know, something like maybe, "Code for ED (Emergency Department or Emergency Medicine), OBS (Observation) and Ambulatory surgery," or something like that.

All I did was code the ICD-9 CM (diagnosis) part. At that time, it was ICD-9. Now, it's ICD-10-CM, part of the test. I didn't code the CPT codes. If you know anything about coding, you know that, I never heard anything back from them and I thought, "Oh my God. I should have coded the CPT codes, but I didn't. I don't know what I was thinking. I guess I wasn't.

I continued to pursue it until I got a job in medical coding. I will say that I did some things to just try and get my foot in the door, such as accept a position as a receptionist, doing some medical records, and then finally passing a test and being able to work as a coder. I just never gave up. As of today, I have been teaching coding for nine or ten years. I have been a Coder/Auditor for sixteen years approximately.

Let's talk about what you should know before you go into coding.

One thing I tell students is this is just like any other job that you would try to get or anything that you would go and try to get a degree for. I really started to equate medical coding to the nursing field and not necessarily because you will take care of patients, per se, but you will have to know a lot about Medical Terminology, Anatomy and Physiology, Disease Process, Drugs and Lab tests.

This could be a catastrophic if you don't know this. I'm speaking truly from experience because I didn't know these things when I first started. I just winged it four or five years or so. It was a real struggle. Of course with ICD-10, it's almost impossible to work if you don't have these fundamental skills.

Chapter 1

Tip 1

Join the Following Groups on LinkedIn. You want to always have your pulse on what is going on in your field. You also want to know what companies are hiring and what other Coders are saying about them.

Join LinkedIn Group-Entry Level Medical Coders

Join LinkedIn Group- Medical Coder

Join LinkedIn Group- Jobs for Medical Coders

Join LinkedIn Group-RHIT & Medical Coding Professionals

Join LinkedIn Group-Remote Medical Coding Professionals

Join LinkedIn Group-Medical Coding

Join LinkedIn Group- Medical Coding Jobs & Training

Join LinkedIn Group- Medical Jobs & Employment

Join LinkedIn Group- Work at Home Medical Coding Job Openings

Join LinkedIn Group-Medical Office (Administrative Assistant/Billing & Coding) NCTC Workgroup

Tip 2

Good grades while you're in school will help you get a job. I get a lot of students that ask me for letters of recommendation- Maybe they haven't worked in a long time. Maybe their employer sent them to get this degree or finish this program so that they can transition from one job to another.

How does it look to ask for letters of recommendation and you made C's in the class? What can the instructor provide in a letter of recommendation for you?

Tip 3

Create a Slide share presentation using your resume. In other words, turn your resume into a PowerPoint Presentation. Go to slide share and LinkedIn for Examples. The key here is use Medical Coding, CPT Coding, CPC (if you are certified), CCS-P (if you have this certification), ICD-10 CM, ICD-10 PCS, any software you used in school particularly Encoder.

Chapter 2

Tip 4

If you want to break into coding, who are your local doctors? Who's your doctor? Who do you see for Cardiology, Family Doctor, Eye Doctor? Who's your dentist? Who's your, if you have children, your pediatrician? Who is your family doctor? If you go see the eye doctor, who's your eye doctor? Who's your OB-GYN, if you're a woman? What doctors do you see on a regular basis?

Do you have a relationship with those doctors or the people in the office, where you can ask if they have an opening? If you go into a clinic for an appointment, ask around. You want to let people know that you're a new coder, and you're looking for any available positions. Let people know that you are available. Your local hospital. Your local doctors.

What you can also do is check the websites of all of the hospitals in your area to see if there's any open positions. You want to just get your foot in the door. If they have anything open in Medical Records or a Coding position, you want to apply, you want to get your name out there so people know that you are looking. As for Local doctors, call the local doctor's offices, ask for an Office Manager, and ask if they're hiring. You can send a blind resume, but I don't recommend that unless you know who to send it to.

Tip 5

Be strategic if you want to get a job when you graduate from school. I advise all of my students to join the AAPC when they start going to school or at least go to all the meetings. Attend as a guest. I think it's $5 to attend as a guest. You can double check that at your local AAPC meeting and that's at AAPC.com. You can see the local chapters, where they meet at, get on their list, or just start going as a visitor. Your school will probably have this information as well.

You can start going to meetings, networking, and find out who the people are that's there. I'm sure you'll find people there that are supervisors. You will find people that are already working in the field. The more you go, you start talking to people, building relationships, you'll be able to get a job once you graduate. For the first couple of meetings, just watch and observe. Of course, if someone ask you who you are be prepared to tell them.

If you're not sure about how to network, you want to read books about networking so you know how to build those relationships. You'll know how to stand out when an employer is looking for a new coder.

Do you know somebody that knows somebody? Who works for a doctor that could tell you if there's an opening, who could put a good word in for you.

I also, recommend that you actually go to the AHIMA local meeting. You can't actually do that unless you're a member of the National AHIMA. You could do that by going to AIHMA.org, and then becoming a member. You can select your local chapter at checkout for an $10. You can create a profile to receive alerts every single day about remote coding positions that they have available. You want to become active in the local chapter. You would do the same thing that you do for AAPC. You just want to meet the people that are there, become active. Of course, if you're a member of AHIMA as well as AAPC you can hold a position, you can volunteer. Learn as much as you can, learn about everyone who is at the meetings. You can do this by Googling their name. Also look them up on LinkedIn and Facebook.

Most people don't know as a medical coder that you have productivity standards, so you have to code so many charts per hour. Then you have accuracy standards as well, which means that maybe, you have to code 8 charts an hour and an accuracy rate of 95%. Some places it's a little bit more. You have to be 95% accurate on the charts that you code, so you really have to know your stuff, and be productive. Accuracy refers to how accurate the CPT codes and ICD-10 CM codes are.

For example, on the inpatient side it is somewhere between 3 or 4 charts per hour depending on length of stay. The production rate for Ambulatory Surgery charts, or Surgery charts is usually 6 to 8 charts per hour. These are the number of charts you would have to code and complete per hour. ED is a little bit more aggressive. If I'm not mistaken, it's somewhere around 20 charts per hour. More on this later.

These are strictly averages. This will vary from hospital to hospital.

Tip 6

The next thing to get or not to get a two-year or four-year degree program. I advise everyone to get an Associate or Bachelor Degree versus a certificate program, unless it's a AAPC program. I do recommend certification programs through AAPC. I am saying if you have a choice between a two year, a four year, or a certificate program, I advise all students to get a two-year degree first, take your certification, get a job, and then go for the four-year degree versus certificate program.

AHIMA offers a comparison here
http://www.ahima.org/careers/plan?tabid=cert .

What I have found is that with the certificate programs, it is a bit harder to get a job. Most companies don't want to hire, or most hospitals don't want to hire students who just receive a certificate. AHIMA has on their website at http://www.ahima.org/careers/codingprograms. Of course, you can try to call AHIMA as well, but they have on their site acceptable two year programs or four year programs. These are acceptable programs that will allow you to sit for certain certification exams such as RHIT (Registered Health Information Technician) and RHIA (Registered Health Information Administrator). RHIA requires a four-year degree from an HIM program accredited by the Commission on Accreditation for Health Informatics and Information Management Education (CAHIIM).

RHIT is a two-year degree from a HIM program accredited by the Commission on Accreditation for Health Informatics and Information Management Education (CAHIIM). You can find out more information at AHIMA.org under Certification.

You can do this online or in person at a brick and mortar school. Most of this is completely online if you want to get a degree. It just makes you more marketable. Most of the time, if you get a two year or four-year degree, you can find a job faster. Whether you get placement or not, the certification will make you a lot more marketable. While you can do this online, in my opinion it is the hardest subject to learn online. It is harder online because you don't know what you don't know. The experience is so much richer in the classroom since you have so many different experiences from other students and so many different questions that others will have that will be so helpful.

Teachers will repeat some of the same things which will help you remember. They will share stories that will also help you remember confusing concepts.

Chapter 3

Tip 7

Google the Temporary Agencies in your Area. Call or go to their website to see if they have any positions available for Medical Coders. The requirements tend to be less stringent which will certainly increase your chances of getting hired. Don't underestimate the power of temporary agencies.

When Employers/Hospitals/Clinics get tired of looking to fill a position they tend to go to a temporary agency. Be sure to call them or check the websites of all temporary agencies websites at least monthly.

Tip 8

Create a Profile on Indeed (www.indeed.com). Sign up for alerts. You will receive job alerts daily. Be sure your profile is complete.

Tip 9

In the beginning, you are a generalist, so you learn all you can about every specialty. You learn all you can about Urology, OB-GYN, Orthopedics, Cardiology, Anesthesia, General Surgery, Observation etc. You learn all you can about the different specialties.

After you get started, and you get your foot in the door wherever you can, you want to start specializing. The money is in the big four. The big four, in my opinion, are Orthopedic, Cardiology, Interventional Radiology, and Inpatient coding. So, these are the four moneymakers. The people that are in these fields make the most money.

You can do this by going to Decision Health. They have a yearly conference on Orthopedic Specialties and Cardiology Specialties. Then, Interventional Radiology, there's a conference for that as well. It's through Z Health Publishing

I mentioned this before, but I'll repeat it here again. Learn all you can about Medical Terminology and Anatomy and Physiology. Once you graduate from school, you want to start taking, especially if you don't get a job right away, you want to start attending webinars through the AAPC as well as the AHIMA.

Chapter 4

Tip 10

It's important that you get certified. When I first started, AAPC was considered the gold standard for Outpatient Coders, but employers tend to side with AHIMA over AAPC even certification wise such as CCS-P over the CPC. I do recommend that you get the CCS-P, which is Certified Coding Specialist Physician-based. Then, the CPC, which is Certified Professional Coder. Both of these certifications is for Outpatient Coders. These are the two main ones if you're just starting off with coding. As a new Coder, you want to stick with Outpatient Coding for at least a couple of years. This depends on where you live, you may need both.

How to make Six Figures as a Medical Coder
Are you a Medical Coder looking to make more money?
Do you want to earn at least $100,000 a year as a Medical Coder?
Are you tired of struggling as a Medical Coder?

Medical Coders are in big demand!

Don't miss the opportunity to get your share of the Medical Coding pie.

This webinar is for you if
- You are a medical Coder
- You want to become a medical Coder
- A seasoned medical coder
- Willing to work hard
- You like to read
- Goal oriented
- Ambitious
- Aggressive

This is not for you if are
- Lazy
- Looking for something quick and easy
- Have no interest in Medical Coding

In this 60-minute webinar you will Learn:
Top Four Paying Coding Areas
What you should be doing as a Coder
Know your worth
Five ways to earn $100,000 or more a year as a Medical Coder

Available on Demand

$99

www.remote-medical-coding-jobs.com

No fluff! Just action packed content for you to take action!

P.S. If you can't attend How to make Six Figures as a Medical Coder live, it will be recorded and you will receive the recording.
P.P.S. You don't want to miss this jam packed Webinar, you won't be sorry. This webinar will be recorded, you can view it anytime. You can watch it as many times as you like.

Tip 11

Post your resume on https://www.aapc.com/memberarea/forums/resume-postings/. You may or may not get any responses. It is still good to have your resume posted here. Also go there periodically and look for openings.

Tip 12

Conduct Informational interviews. If you're serious about becoming a medical coder, as soon as you can, you want to start doing Informational interviews. What you want to do is call the HIM department of hospitals. You will want to speak with the HIM Director. If it is a doctor's office, you will want to speak with the Office Manager.

You just want to talk to them about how you can get started in coding, what recommendations they have, what do they look for in coders, and you really want to put yourself on the radar for them to start thinking about you when you graduate. Always send a thank you letter or thank you card after the informational interview. Ask good questions, research the hospital, learn the requirements, this will help you in the future. You won't ask basic questions that you can find on the internet. A few questions you could ask is Do you hire New Coders? What do you look for when hiring new graduates?

Chapter 5

Tip 13

Know the ICD-10-CM coding guidelines. The coding guidelines can be found at the beginning of your ICD-10 CM manual. This can be a downfall for some coders because they don't like to read and so they don't read the guidelines. This is so important. FYI, if you don't like to read, then coding may not be for you because there's a lot of reading, there's a lot of research, there's a lot of digging.

You don't have to memorize them. You just need to be very familiar with them.

Tip 14

The next thing is it costs a little bit of money to be a Medical Coder. Depending on what company you get hired with, sometimes you don't get hired right away -maybe it'll take a month or two. You have to pay for your webinars, conferences, memberships etc,. This is probably already paid for through your school, but you might have AAPC dues if you want join and your school didn't pay. You might have to buy manuals, ICD-10 CM manual, the CPT manual. You might have AHIMA dues or you might pay for AHIMA webinars or AAPC webinars.

Don't worry too much because more than likely when you get a job, your employer will pay for all of this or at least the majority of it.

Tip 15

Look for non-coding HIM jobs, for example Registration, Account Rep, Claim Follow up, Charge Entry, etc. You want something to get your foot in the door, gain experience (daily use of ICD 10-CM and CPT) and then move up to a coding job.

Chapter 6

Tip 16

Pay attention to the demand in your area. Before you graduate, you want to make sure that you've been looking at the AAPC website, looking at Indeed.com, looking at your newspaper for jobs that are in the employment section of your newspaper. You should also look at Monster.com or CareerBuilder in your area to see what jobs are in demand. Of course, if you work remote, you can work anywhere in the country and you want to see what specialties are in demand.

Tip 17

Apply for a PFS (Patient Financial Services) position or Collections. The company that hire you will train you. This makes it easy to get your foot in the door. Working for a Hospital in this position is a great start.

Tip 18

Complete a LinkedIn profile. You would go to LinkedIn.com, if you don't have a profile, create one. You want to make sure each field is completed. You want to use the keywords: medical coder and if you have certifications you want to put those in your profile as well. These keywords will come up when recruiters are looking for people. Make sure you have Medical Coder/Medical Coding in your Headline, Summary, Skills and Expertise. Even if you have to put Future Medical Coder or Medical Coding Graduate/Student.

Chapter 7 Cover Letters

Always write a cover letter for any job you are applying to. Keep Cover Letter to one page. This is one of the most neglected things by most job applicants. This is important as it will make you stand out. It takes time but it's super easy.

What you want to do is pull from the requirements of the job and match up with your experience so the employer knows that you have this experience. You can still do this even if you don't have any experience. Be sure to use any software you used in your Classes. Other keywords you should use is CPT, HCPCS, ICD-10-CM. You would have used these as a bare minimum in class.

Also when you're reviewing the requirements of a job you want to pull those key words out and put them in your resume, whether it's under your skills section or qualifications section. You want to pull those key words out and put them in your resume. Especially in your resume, but also on your cover letter as well.

The reason why it's so important to pull the key words from the job requirements and put into your resume is because most applications now are done electronically.

Part of the reason why is because technology is changing so fast. It's also because the number of applicants that are applying for jobs used to be a dozen or so, now it could be in the hundreds.

The way employers rule you out is by using these keywords. They have a filter that says, "These key words don't show up in this person's resume, and then you are weeded out." Even though you might be qualified to do the job. You want to make sure that you're using the key words pulled directly from the job description or job posting to get through the job filters.

1234 ABC Street   (123) 456-7890
Dream Job, USA 45678   professionalemail@yahoo.com

October 21, 2013

Name of person resume is going to if known

His or her title

Name of company

Address

City, State Zip

To Whom It May Concern:

My 15 plus years' experience in Medical Billing, Coding, and Auditing makes me a great candidate for the Remote coding position.

My qualifications include:

- Certified Coding Specialist (CCS) Keywords employer is looking for
- 4 years' experience as Auditor
- 13 years coding Physician Services
- ICD-10 training
- 1995 and 1997 guidelines experience
- 8 years coding for a teaching hospital
- Executive Masters of Business Administration

- 10 years Management Experience, Previous experience as CEO/President
- Taught classes at Remington College in Professional Development, Medical Coding, Medical Billing, Anatomy and Physiology
- Teach Medical Coding and Billing at Online School

I am committed to the coding field, and I am focused on accuracy. I look forward to speaking with you about this opportunity.

Thank you for your time and consideration.

Sincerely,

Jane Doe, MBA, CCS, CCS-P, CPC (Any Certifications if applicable, higher degrees)

Enclosure: Resume

Chapter 8 Resume

Keep Resume to 2 pages or less. Use a different resume for each job you apply to by making subtle tweaks as needed. Be sure to save under that Job title on your computer. Companies sometimes call the same job something different based on Employer. Check your resume for spelling and grammatical errors. This is a big no-no, and this happens more frequently than not. If you've looked at your resume several times, maybe you need a fresh set of eyes on it. Of course, Microsoft Word has tried to do their best to offer the red and green squiggly lines for spelling and grammatical errors, but you might just get a fresh set of eyes and get someone else to look at it for you.

Take off work older than 10 years or older unless you have been with your current employer longer than 10 years. In other words, you want at least 2 previous jobs besides where you are currently, if applicable. You don't won't to use jobs you had in high school if you are in your 30s.

When you have jobs on your resume that you've done in the past, you want to make sure that you have added the -ed indicating that they were in the past. When you look at your resume you know, for example, if I filed last year, then I'd do "filed" with an -ed versus "file", because file will indicate that I'm doing it presently.

Google Resumes for the Job you are searching for and your industry as well.

Make sure your email is a professional one.

Core Competencies should be keywords taken directly from the Job description that match your experience.

Always spell check all documents.

Don't include months on your resume especially if you are trying to cover up short periods of time.

Your Name, MBA, CCS, CCS-P, CPC

1234 Going Places Dr	(123) 456-7809
Going Places, USA 12345	professionalemail@yahoo.com

OUTPATIENT MEDICAL CODER

EDUCATION

Certified Coding Specialist (CCS)   2012

  AHIMA

Certified Coding Specialist-Physician   2012

(CCS-P)

  AHIMA

Certified Professional Coder   2009

(CPC)

  American Academy of Professional Coders (AAPC)

Executive Masters of Business Administration

Colorado Technical University,   2007

Colorado Springs, CO

Bachelor of Science, Business Administration

Colorado Technical University, Colorado   2006

Springs, CO

Magna Cum Laude GPA 3.7

Medical Office Specialist

American School of Business   2000

CORE COMPETENCIES Your Industry Keywords that match your experience

ASC/SDS/OBS/ED	MS-DRG
APC	ICD-10 PCS
RAC/CERT	Auditing
EPIC/Centricity	Intelicode Pro
Citrix/NextGen	3M/Encoder Pro
IDX	Interventional Radiology
Home Health/Nursing Home	Clinical Documentation Improvement
POAs/HACs	MPFS/RVU's
Meditech	Level 1 Trauma
Clintrac	PowerChart
Canopy	ChartOne/ewebhealth
HDM/Citrix	TruCode
VPNs	Sovera
Sunrise	Affinity
Quantim	ICD-10 CM

PROFESSIONAL EXPERIENCE

Kingsley Rose   2015-present

REMOTE CODER/AUDITOR

- Analyzed and interpreted inpatient, medical records to ensure complete and accurate coding based on ICD-9 Coding Guidelines and UHDDS
- Coded all pertinent comorbid and complications as well as invasive procedures
- Validated discharge disposition code assignment
- Coded all diagnostic and operative information from the medical record using ICD-9-CM, CPT and HCPCS coding classification systems

PREVIOUS EXPERIENCE

Willis Knighton Health System   2001-2003

(250 bed, nonprofit)

INPATIENT/OUTPATIENT MEDICAL CODER

- Coded all pertinent comorbid and complications as well as invasive procedures
- Responsible for assigning ICD-9, CPT-4 codes to obtain accurate DRG or APC assignment for proper reimbursement and data collection

- Assigned POA (Present on Admission) indicators per official guidelines
- Validate discharge disposition code assignment

Professional Associations

AHIMA	2012-present
ACIDS	2012-present
AAPC	2009-present

Chapter 9 A Word on Remote Coding

I advise all coders, or potential coders, to start talking to other coders, find out what their experiences are, what they're going through, what challenges they're dealing with, what they like, what they don't like.

Coder's especially new coders need a support group. Coding from home can be a lonely experience. You need to have someone you can call if you need help. It might be you just need a break or you might have a coding question.

Remote Coding is lonely. It is hard. You have to build a network of coders, of people, you can trust and call when you need help. Be aware when you take a test for a firm, sometimes the people who grade the test are usually coders and may not know what they are doing.

When you are a Remote Coder, there is the client or the hospital and the firm or the Agency (Recruiter). Keep in mind the client (hospital) holds all the cards. They can cancel a project at a moment's notice and they often do. To the agency, the client is the most important. I'm sure you understand since the money comes from the client.

Disadvantages

- A project can be canceled at a moment's notice. Projects can last 4 weeks or 4 years.

- No benefits-depends on who you work for and whether you are full or part time.

Remote coding is a lot of hurry up and wait. Clients cancel and delay projects all the time. You will have to wait usually 1 to 3 weeks maybe longer for paperwork and IT access. This is normal and happens usually with every project. You are at the beck and call of the client.

The road for a coder is long and hard. I get a lot of students that tell me, that they want to do medical coding because they heard that it was easy. They can stay home. They can take care of their kids. They can do whatever they want and have a flexible schedule. This is a myth in a sense.

Yes, you can work from home, but you need to really bring your A game. You really need to be very knowledgeable about Coding. You need to learn everything that you can so that when you're at home, you can figure things out. You have to have good research skills. You have to be able to figure things out on your own that maybe you don't know. So, it's not easy. You have to be detail oriented. You have to be very analytical.

What I found is that I've worked remote for 6 years and people don't respect your time when you work from home. It could be a blessing and a curse. You find yourself really having a flexible schedule. You can do what you want and you tend to run around, do your errands during the day. Things that you would normally do after work, you can now do those during the day. You don't have to ask anybody if you want to go take your child to the doctor or if you want to go to the doctor.

It's a balancing act. It's not just being able to do what you want to. You still have to come back home and make up those hours.

Before you start another project

Consider the following

Is the agency offering benefits?

W2 employee or 1099 (W2 is usually better) (1099 employees don't have taxes taken out. You will have to itemize taxes for it to be beneficial. Benefits are limited with 1099)

401k

Continuing education

Books-Do they provide new books each year?

PTO/sick time/Holiday Pay Do you get it?

Does the hospital use Quadramed? Quadramed is a pain in the butt for me.

Does the hospital use handwritten record? Will the records you will be coding handwritten? (While most records will be electronic, you could have handwritten records scanned into the medical record.)

Will your schedule be flexible or a strict schedule (daytime hours or 8-5)? What time zone is client?

How much are you willing to accept per hour?

Productivity

This depends on the hospital.

ER (Emergency Department) 12-20 charts per hour

SDS (Same Day Surgery) 6-8 charts per hour

Inpatient 2 to 3 per hour (While this is the normal 24 to 25 is expected per day)

Diagnostic Varies usually over 200

Chapter 10 Learning is Key

Learn all you can while you're in school. In other words, I find students who rush through school just to try to finish so they can get a job. They just want to get through. They just want it done. This is totally understandable but this will be detrimental to their career.

To me this is a terrible thing to do because, while you can rush it and get through (the Medical Coding Program) and study enough to pass the test and make an A. This is horrible when it comes to actually working as a Medical Coder. You don't know medical terminology. Medical Terminology is a foundation skill. You don't know key words that will help you do your job on a daily basis. You don't know why patients have XYZ. Anatomy & Physiology is crucial.

It's so fundamental that you learn everything you can about Medical Terminology, Anatomy and Physiology, Disease process, Drugs and Lab Tests. I speak from three points of view if you will. I have seen Inpatient and Outpatient Coders struggle (I had to audit them), I've been an Inpatient and an Outpatient Coder and I speak as someone who didn't learn myself. I see it as an instructor as well. I would have to say that Inpatient is harder especially if you don't know these things.

For Outpatient Coders, you will need to know Medical Terminology and Anatomy and Physiology more so than the others. These other things if you know them, Disease Processes, Drugs, Lab Tests, they would be beneficial bonuses.

Outpatient Test Areas

Whenever you want to get a job as a medical coder, no matter if it's remote or not, you will have to pass a test. What I mean by "remote" is you work from home and maybe the hospital that you work for or, the recruitment company, maybe they're in another state. You still will have to take a test in order to get the job. A coding assessment is what they call it. You might receive a word document or a PDF file that you will have to complete. You have to pass the test in order to get the job.

Some companies have, an electronic version of the test. So, you would sign in to a secure website and you will get two hours or four hours to take the test approximately.

Since the inception of ICD-10 CM it is best to know the ICD-10-CM Coding guidelines. It is also helpful to read instructions/notes above and below the code.

Most Remote Coders work multiple contracts. Coders work multiple contracts due to the fact one day you can be working, the next you might not. Of course, there are Permanent Contracts. The pay tends to be lower but they will provide you with PTO, Benefits, etc.

Remote Coders also work more than one contract to make more money. I don't know any remote coders who only work 1 contract.

Typically, Remote Coders can earn anywhere from $22-$65 per hour. It is important to know how much you will work for. You will get this question all the time. Take into consideration the whole package-benefits, PTO, 401k and flexibility.

What you have to realize is even if a contract ends the recruiter and the agency still get paid from other contracts where as you won't if a contract ends. Always keep this in mind. This is the worst thing being a Remote Coder is getting a check one day and the next day not getting one. Make sure you protect yourself.

Remote Coders have to be the fastest and the most accurate to continue working. This is necessary since with each new contract, you will be audited within the first month.

Remote Coders should be (it would be helpful to have)

- The highest Internet speed in your area
- Dual Screens (makes you faster)
- ICD-10-CM Coding Book (Current Year)
- Abbreviation Book (Use Google)
- Coding Clinic (AHA-American Hospital Association)
- Clinical Coding Workout with Answers (AHIMA Product)

- Basic Knowledge of all Specialties
- Some knowledge of Billing
- Medicare Website
- MS-DRG Expert Book (Current Year) (even if you code Outpatient only)
- Edits (It is important to know how to work edits)
- SOI (Severity of Illness)
- Excel on your computer
- Medical Dictionary (Use Google)
- A & P Book (Use Google)
- Scratch paper
- Pen
- Sticky notes
- Tabs for your book

Remote Coders

- Become the best
- Know your ICD-10 CM Coding Guidelines
- Get the experience even if you work for peanuts at first
- Read your AAPC magazine and the AHIMA Journal (Become a member if you are not already).
- Pay for Webinars-learn all you can (Decision Health, AAPC, AHIMA, Z-Health Publishing).

- Attend AAPC and AHIMA Conferences.
- Participate in round tables. (Check with your Local AHIMA).
- Study trends (What's new in healthcare).
- Attend local meetings for AAPC and AHIMA (National and Regional).
- Become a Speaker at a Conference (National or Regional AAPC/AHIMA).
- Focus on a Niche in a hard area like Cardiology/ Orthopedics/ Anesthesia/ Auditing/ Interventional Radiology/ Inpatient Coding (see the resource section).
- Go the extra mile.
- Learn about Compliance/Auditing.
- Join AHIMA/AAPC if you haven't already
- Get Certified CPC, CCS-P, CCS, CPC-H etc
- Give value for what you are paid (Work all the time you are working)
- Commit to becoming more accurate and more productive (Learn from your Audits)

Take medical terminology as your foundation and learn all you can from it. Medical terminology is hard. It's like a new language. It's different. It's something that we're not used to. Don't just skate by memorizing the terms and then forgetting them after the test. Take the time to really learn the terms.

I think that this is so important. You have to learn as many words as you can. This is vital if you want to be successful as a Medical Coder. You need to make sure that you learn medical terminology.

Read Coding clinics. This is produced by the AHA (American Hospital Association). This really gives you tips about how to code something. This is mostly the ICD-10-CM and the ICD-PCS (Inpatient Coding). There is also the CPT assistant (AMA-American Medical Association) for the CPT coding.

So, you have the coding clinic for the ICD-10 CM as well as the ICD-10 PCS. Then you have the CPT assistant for the CPT side, or the Physician based.

If you like to read a lot, then Ambulatory Surgery or Inpatient Coding, might be for you. I don't recommend Inpatient Coding for beginners, so I will just say if you like to read a lot, then Ambulatory Surgery may be for you.

The last thing is practice, practice, practice. If you're a coder, you went to school for coding or you're in school to be a coder, you want to practice as much as you can. If you miss something, you want to go in reverse and figure out why you missed that code. That's really the only way that you learn. You just backtrack and then you see, "Okay, why did I miss this? How did I miss this? How did I get the wrong code?" You start with the correct code given. You read the description and then you start from the Index and determine what they choose as the main term etc.

Make sure that you read the notes above and below the codes. Sometimes that'll let you know what you missed or why you missed it.

The cost and investment are similar to that of a nurse, because nurses have to get CEUs and medical coders have to get CEUs as well. You will attend webinars or conferences to receive those CEUs. If you want to be the best you will have to take education very seriously. You can also build great relationships as well as have people to call on when you have a Coding dilemma.

You will feel like a doctor when it's all said and done. Sometimes you have to read between the lines. Sometimes you have to figure out, especially with the new changes in ICD-10, you have to figure out what the doctor is trying to tell us.

Chapter 11 Remote Coding Hiring Process

Most jobs require 2 to 3 year's experience. If you have the experience, you will send your resume. If they are interested, most companies will interview you. Some will test you first and follow it up with an interview. The recruiter will send your resume to client. They (the client-hospital) may call you. You get hired or feedback. They may test you even if you take a test for the Company you are working for. If hired, you will complete paperwork/application/IT Paperwork.

Be sure to start with doctors that you currently see for your healthcare needs such as Family Doctor, Pediatrician, and Cardiologist etc. Ask them if they have openings. Also check your local hospital for openings. Consider taking a position just to get your foot in the door such as Medical Records position. It is important to do Information Interviews here to increase your chances of being hired. It is also necessary to attend your local AAPC meetings. This will also increase your chances of being hired. Focus on building relationships and learning all you can at the AAPC meetings.

Common Questions a Hospital may ask (Have your resume in front of you)

- Systems you've used
- Cases you've coded

- Productivity
- Last QA Scores
- Areas you've coded in
- They may ask you specific Coding Questions
- Always have your CPT (Outpatient) and ICD-10 CM book especially for Inpatient
- Hospitals you've worked for

You should have questions to ask the Client as well such as the Encoder they used, Productivity Standard, and Potential Start Date, How soon they plan to hire someone. Is this Temporary or Permanent?

Research Hospital before call

Ask Recruiter Questions about the hospital as well as the person who will be calling you or that you will call. You want any information they have.

Salaries

"Opportunities continue to abound as HIM departments across the U.S. expand their staffs to help complete the transition to ICD-10 coding, perform data analytics, protect patient data and prevent data breaches. All of which translated to an average salary that was 11% higher than last year, at $61,005 for all survey takers."

Remote Coding Companies

Himagine

Precyse

CSI

Altegra

Harmony Healthcare

Kindred Health

Comforce

HCTec

Workbeast

Maxim

UASI

Codebusters

Thor Group

LexiCode

Oxford HIM

Appendix A

Books I recommend for studying

ICD-10-CM and ICD-10 PCS Coding Handbook (Current Year) with Answers

ICD-10-PCS An Applied Approach AHIMA Current Year

DRG Expert Current Year

Clinical Coding Workout with Answers Current Year

Current Year CDI Pocket Guide (HCMarketplace.com)

AAPC offers Books on Specialties to study for Certifications but they are good for studying the specialty along with CPT guidelines.

Appendix B

Resources

Advance Healthcare Network

AAPC

AHIMA

Decision Health

Certification Coaching Org cco.us Free webinar monthly with free CEUs

Libman Education (www.libmaneducation.com)

To learn more about Ambulatory Surgery Coding go to

https://www.cms.gov/Center/Provider-Type/Ambulatory-Surgical-Centers-ASC-Center.html

To learn more about Evaluation and Management Coding and how you will be audited

https://www.cms.gov/outreach-and-education/medicare-learning-network-MLN/MLNedwebguide/emdoc.html

To check a code for medical necessity

https://www.cms.gov/Research-Statistics-Data-and-Systems/Monitoring-Programs/Medicare-FFS-Compliance-Programs/Medical-Review/

https://www.cms.gov/Regulations-and-Guidance/Legislation/CLIA/index.html

To help you work OPPS edits
https://www.cms.gov/Medicare/Coding/OutpatientCodeEdit/Downloads/DetailedOPPSProgramEdits.pdf

Before You Leave

I need your help. When you go to the next page, Kindle gives you an opportunity to share your thoughts and opinions through your Facebook and Twitter account. If you believe your friends and family will benefit from this book, please share your thoughts with them. You might change someone's life, and I would be eternally grateful to you.

If you feel strongly about the contributions this book made to your life, please take a few seconds to post a 5-star review on Amazon. Very few people ever leave 5 star review. So it is a big deal if you do. Writing a 5-star review is like tipping me $25. I really appreciate the gesture. I feel like a million bucks whenever I get a glowing review.

If you have any questions, you can reach me via Shondamiles@yahoo.com. I will try to respond to your questions as soon as possible. You can also connect with me on Facebook and Twitter.

How to make Six Figures as a Medical Coder

Are you a Medical Coder looking to make more money?
Do you want to earn at least $100,000 a year as a Medical Coder?
Are you tired of struggling as a Medical Coder?

Medical Coders are in big demand!

Don't miss the opportunity to get your share of the Medical Coding pie.

This webinar is for you if
- You are a medical Coder
- You want to become a medical Coder
- A seasoned medical coder
- Willing to work hard
- You like to read
- Goal oriented
- Ambitious
- Aggressive

This is not for you if are
- Lazy
- Looking for something quick and easy
- Have no interest in Medical Coding

In this 60-minute webinar you will Learn:
Top Four Paying Coding Areas
What you should be doing as a Coder
Know your worth
Five ways to earn $100,000 or more a year as a Medical Coder

Available on Demand

$99

www.remote-medical-coding-jobs.com

No fluff! Just action packed content for you to take action!

P.S. If you can't attend How to make Six Figures as a Medical Coder live, it will be recorded and you will receive the recording.
P.P.S. You don't want to miss this jam packed Webinar, you won't be sorry. This webinar will be recorded, you can view it anytime. You can watch it as many times as you like.

About the Author

Shonda Miles has been self-employed for 18 years. She has owned businesses ranging from an online retail store to a Training Company.

Shonda Miles is the CEO of Shonda Miles International, a company helping organizations and individuals improve performance and achieve their goals. Shonda Miles is here to help you achieve your full potential. Her purpose is to help millions of people achieve their goals and live their God given talent.

Shonda Miles is an Author, Entrepreneur, Speaker, Personal Development Trainer, Business Consultant and Business Coach. She loves reading Nonfiction books, writing business books and shopping. Personal Development is her mission. Shonda speaks, blogs and writes about a variety of personal development topics such as Time Management, Success, Goal Setting and having a Positive Attitude.

Shonda's goal is to help others achieve the level of success they desire.

Shonda Miles is a MBA Graduate. She has several successful businesses.

Shonda Miles can be reached at www.remote-medical-coding-jobs.com or by email at info@remote-medical-coding-jobs.com

62020323R00033

Made in the USA
Middletown, DE
17 January 2018